170+ PALEO FOODS FOR BEGINNERS

+ FREE PALEO DIET RECIPES

BY

TREASURE JULIUS

TABLE OF CONTENTS

INTRODUCTION TO PALEO DIET

What is the Paleo Diet?

The paleo diet, also known as the Paleolithic diet or the caveman diet, is a popular dietary approach that attempts to mimic the eating habits of early humans during the Paleolithic era. Proponents of the paleo diet believe that our bodies are genetically adapted to the diet of our Paleolithic ancestors and that modern agricultural practices and processed foods have led to various health problems.

The core idea behind the paleo diet is to eat foods that were available to our hunter-gatherer ancestors, such as:

1. Lean meats: Preferably from animals that were grass-fed or wild game.
2. Fish: Especially those rich in omega-3 fatty acids, like salmon.
3. Fruits and vegetables: Except for starchy vegetables like potatoes.
4. Nuts and seeds: Except for peanuts which are legumes.
5. Healthy fats: Such as olive oil, coconut oil, and avocado oil.
6. Avoiding processed foods: This includes refined sugars, grains, and most dairy products.

Foods to be avoided in the paleo diet typically include:

1. Grains: Including wheat, oats, and barley.
2. Legumes: Such as beans, lentils, and peanuts.
3. Dairy: Except for some versions of the paleo diet that include certain dairy products like butter or ghee.
4. Processed foods: Including refined sugars, artificial sweeteners, and most packaged foods.

The paleo diet encourages the consumption of whole, unprocessed foods while eliminating grains, legumes, and dairy. Advocates of the diet claim it can lead to weight loss, improved energy levels, and better overall health. However, it's essential to note that the scientific community's opinions on the paleo diet are mixed, and individual results may vary. Before making significant changes to your diet, it's always a good idea to consult with a healthcare provider or a registered dietitian.

2.5 million years ago, the early man foraged and hunted for seafood, meat, vegetables, fruit, nuts, roots and seeds. This period of time before the development of agriculture is known as the Paleolithic era. The Paleo diet is also known as the Stone Age diet, hunter gathering diet and the caveman diet. No matter what you call our ancestors, some things haven't changed. Man's digestive systems have evolved only the slightest amount in the 10,000 years since farming changed our diets. Shortened to Paleo, the modern diet is an approach to nutrition that mimics the early man's diet for ultimate health.

Our minds are modern, but our bodies and brains still need the same food.

Gastroenterologist Walter L. Voegtlin first popularized the Paleo diet in the 1970's. He argued in, "The Stone Age Diet," humans as carnivores, chiefly needs fats, proteins and a small amount of carbohydrates for optimum performance. For the last 30 years, obesity has been increasing in the United States. Our modern diets are laden with preservatives, processed

sugars, and fried foods. Today's health crisis has led to a renewed interest in Voegtlin's tested approach to healthy living.

Benefits of the Paleo Diet

The advantages of the Paleo Diet have been researched and proven in numerous academic journals. It is amazing how changing what we put in our mouths can cause dramatic changes in our quality of life.

o Lose fat- Though the Paleo diet is designed as a weight loss plan people inherently lose weight. The foods that make up the Paleo diet are what we call fat burning foods. In fact, the Paleo diet allows you to eat large quantities of delicious food while restricting calories. The result is a lean, fit body.

The paleo diet, also known as the Paleolithic diet or caveman diet, is based on the presumed ancient diet of our ancestors who lived during the Paleolithic era, which lasted around 2.5 million to 10,000 years ago. The diet emphasizes whole foods, lean proteins, fruits, vegetables, nuts, and seeds, while avoiding processed foods, grains, legumes, dairy, and refined sugars. Advocates of the paleo diet claim several potential benefits:

1. Weight Loss: Many people adopt the paleo diet to lose weight. By avoiding processed foods and sugars, individuals may naturally reduce their calorie intake and lose weight.

2. Improved Blood Sugar Levels: The diet's focus on whole foods and avoidance of refined sugars and grains can help stabilize blood sugar levels, which is beneficial for individuals with diabetes or those at risk of developing diabetes.

3. Better Digestive Health: Eliminating grains and legumes might be helpful for people with certain digestive issues like irritable bowel syndrome (IBS) or gluten sensitivity, although this varies from person to person.

4. Increased Nutrient Intake: By emphasizing whole foods, the paleo diet can increase the intake of essential nutrients such as vitamins, minerals, and antioxidants.

5. Higher Protein Intake: The paleo diet encourages the consumption of lean meats and fish, which are excellent sources of high-quality protein. Protein is essential for muscle repair and growth, as well as for maintaining a healthy immune system.

6. Reduced Inflammation: Some proponents of the paleo diet suggest that it can help reduce inflammation in the body, which is believed to be a factor in various chronic diseases.

7. Improved Energy Levels: By avoiding processed foods and focusing on nutrient-dense whole foods, some people report having more stable energy levels throughout the day.

8. Better Skin Health: For some individuals, eliminating dairy and processed foods might lead to clearer skin and a reduction in conditions like acne or eczema.

9. Enhanced Mental Clarity: Some people claim that following a paleo diet improves mental clarity and focus. However, scientific evidence supporting this claim is limited.

It's important to note that while some individuals may experience these benefits, the paleo diet is not without controversy. Critics argue that it can be restrictive, making it difficult for some people to sustain in the long term. Additionally, the evolutionary basis of the diet has been challenged, and the diet's impact on cardiovascular health due to its emphasis on high-fat animal products is a topic of ongoing research and debate.

As with any diet, it's advisable to consult with a healthcare provider or a registered dietitian before making significant changes to your eating habits, especially if you have underlying health conditions.

o Fight Disease- The Paleo diet is proven to help prevent diabetes, Parkinson's avoid Parkinson's, cancer, heart disease and strokes.

o Improve Digestion- Many digestive problems such as, irritable bowel syndrome, Crohn's disease and indigestion can be avoided.

o Combats Acne– Eating the Paleo way means avoiding the foods that cause acne. When sebum is overproduced or obstructed the sebaceous glands enlarge and form pimples. Foods in the Paleo diet do not cause the insulin spikes that cause a sebum boost. As a result, you can expect smoother, more attractive skin.

o Feel Good- Not only does the Paleo diet help people healthier and look younger it also makes you feel better. Paleo supporters swear by the caveman lifestyle because it just "feels" right. The only way to find out the energy and confidence they experience is to try it for yourself.

DIETING THE PALEO WAY

Diet Basics

People assume the Paleo Diet is complicated and difficult to follow. It is actually quite simple. Eat real foods. For a guideline on portions, 56–65% of your calories should come from animals, 36–45% from plant based foods. Keep proteins high at 19-35% carbohydrates at 22-40% and fat at 28-58%.

PALEO DIET

Following the Paleo diet involves eating foods that our ancestors from the Paleolithic era would have consumed. The idea is to focus on whole, unprocessed foods and avoid modern processed foods. Here are the basic principles of the Paleo diet:

Foods to Eat:

1. Lean Proteins: Including beef, pork, poultry, fish, seafood, and eggs. Opt for grass-fed, free-range, or wild-caught options whenever possible.

2. Fruits: All kinds of fruits, preferably fresh and in season.

3. Vegetables: All types of vegetables are allowed, both cooked and raw.

4. Nuts and Seeds: Such as almonds, walnuts, flaxseeds, and chia seeds.

5. Healthy Fats: Avocado, olive oil, coconut oil, and animal fats from grass-fed sources.

6. Tubers: Such as sweet potatoes and other root vegetables.

7. Herbs and Spices: Use various herbs and spices to add flavor to your dishes.

Eating a Paleo Diet is more about experimenting than limitations. Mother Nature provides a large variety of delicious foods to explore. Instead of settling for a box of processed macaroni and cheese, feast on a meal that excites your taste buds and your energy level. Here is a small list of the many foods to incorporate into your diet.

PROTEINS

Beef

Pheasant

Goose

Tuna

Lobster

Chicken eggs

Veal

Deer

Chicken

Salmon

Shrimp

Goose eggs

Pork

Duck

Turkey

Trout

Scallops

Duck eggs

Lamb

Wild Turkey Quail

Halibut

Crab

Quail eggs

Goat

Rabbit

Duck

Sole

Clams

VEGETABLES

Cauliflower

Collard Greens

Butternut

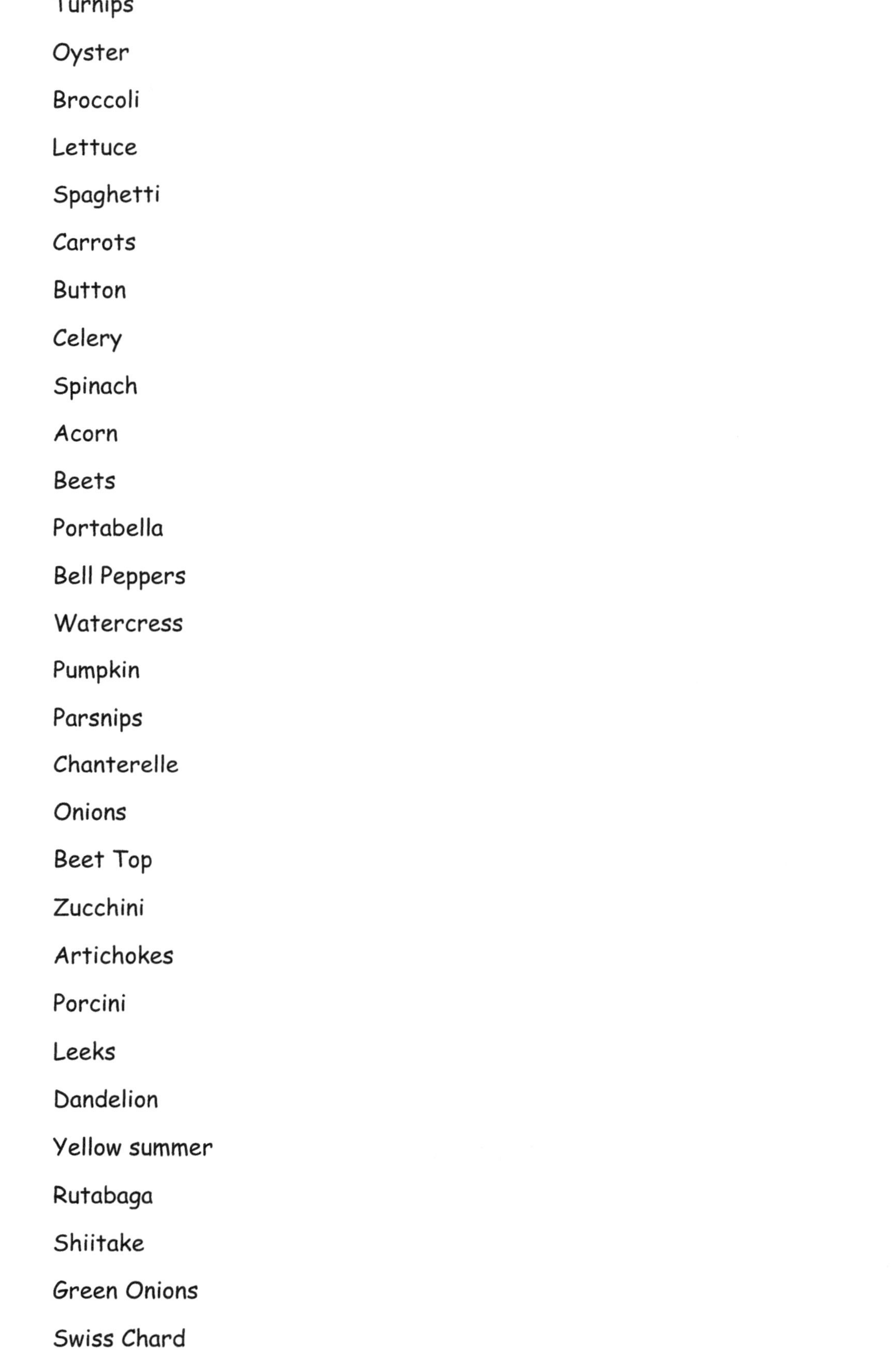

Turnips

Oyster

Broccoli

Lettuce

Spaghetti

Carrots

Button

Celery

Spinach

Acorn

Beets

Portabella

Bell Peppers

Watercress

Pumpkin

Parsnips

Chanterelle

Onions

Beet Top

Zucchini

Artichokes

Porcini

Leeks

Dandelion

Yellow summer

Rutabaga

Shiitake

Green Onions

Swiss Chard

Buttercup

Sweet Potatoes

Crimini

Eggplant

Mustard Greens

Crookneck

Radish

Morel

Brussels Sprout

Kale

Yams

Artichokes

Turnip Greens

Cassava

Asparagus

Seaweed

Cucumber

Endive

Cabbage

Arugula

Okra

Avocados

SUPPORTING PLAYERS

Olive Oil

Apples

Brazil Nuts

Cayenne Pepper

Parsley

Avocado

Oranges

Pistachios

Chilies

Thyme

Coconut Oil

Bananas

Sunflower

Seeds

Ginger

Lavender

Rabbit

Moose

Bass

Mussels

Sheep

Woodcock

Haddock

Oysters

Wild Boar

Elk

Turbot

Bison

Cod

Tilapia

Walleye

Flatfish

Grouper

Mackerel

Herring

Anchovy

Clarified Butter

Strawberry

Pumpkin Seeds

Onions

Mint

Lard

Cranberry

Sesame Seeds

Garlic

Rosemary

Tallow

Grapefruit

Pecans

Black Pepper

Chives

Veal Fat

Peaches

Walnuts

Hot Peppers

Tarragon

Duck Fat

Pears

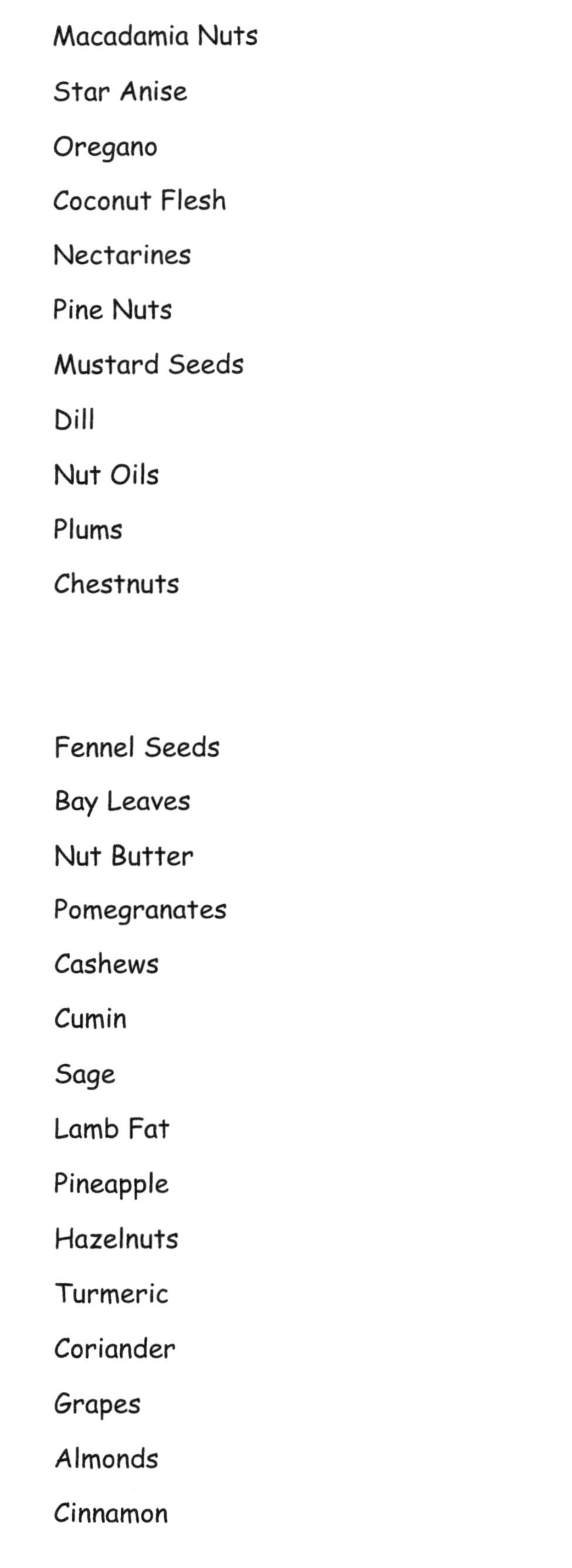

Macadamia Nuts

Star Anise

Oregano

Coconut Flesh

Nectarines

Pine Nuts

Mustard Seeds

Dill

Nut Oils

Plums

Chestnuts

Fennel Seeds

Bay Leaves

Nut Butter

Pomegranates

Cashews

Cumin

Sage

Lamb Fat

Pineapple

Hazelnuts

Turmeric

Coriander

Grapes

Almonds

Cinnamon

Papaya

Paprika

Cantaloupe

Nutmeg

Kiwi

Cloves

Lychee

Vanilla

Paleo recipes

Here are three delicious Paleo diet recipes you can try:

1. Paleo Grilled Chicken with Vegetables

 Ingredients:
- 2 boneless, skinless chicken breasts
- 2 tablespoons olive oil
- 1 teaspoon paprika
- 1 teaspoon garlic powder
- Salt and pepper to taste
- Assorted vegetables (bell peppers, zucchini, mushrooms), sliced
- Fresh herbs (rosemary, thyme) for garnish

 Instructions:
1. Preheat your grill or grill pan over medium-high heat.

2. In a small bowl, mix olive oil, paprika, garlic powder, salt, and pepper.

3. Brush the chicken breasts and vegetables with the olive oil mixture.

4. Grill the chicken for 6-7 minutes per side or until cooked through (internal temperature of 165°F/74°C). Grill the vegetables until they are tender and slightly charred.

5. Remove from the grill and let the chicken rest for a few minutes before slicing.

6. Serve the grilled chicken and vegetables, garnished with fresh herbs.

2. Paleo Cauliflower Fried Rice

Ingredients:
- 1 head cauliflower, grated into rice-like texture
- 2 tablespoons coconut oil
- 2 cloves garlic, minced
- 1 small onion, finely chopped
- 1 carrot, diced
- 1 cup frozen peas and carrots, thawed
- 2 eggs, beaten
- 3 tablespoons coconut aminos (Paleo-friendly soy sauce alternative)
- Salt and pepper to taste
- Green onions, chopped, for garnish

Instructions:
1. Heat coconut oil in a large skillet or wok over medium heat.

2. Add garlic and onion, sauté until translucent.

3. Add diced carrot and cook until slightly tender.

4. Push the vegetables to one side of the pan and pour the beaten eggs into the other side. Scramble the eggs until fully cooked, then mix with the vegetables.

5. Add grated cauliflower to the pan. Stir in the peas, carrots, and coconut aminos.

6. Cook for 5-7 minutes, stirring frequently until the cauliflower is tender.

7. Season with salt and pepper. Garnish with chopped green onions before serving.

3. Paleo Baked Salmon with Lemon and Dill

Ingredients:
- 2 salmon fillets
- 2 tablespoons olive oil
- 1 lemon, thinly sliced
- 2 tablespoons fresh dill, chopped
- Salt and pepper to taste

Instructions:
1. Preheat the oven to 375°F (190°C).
2. Place the salmon fillets on a baking sheet lined with parchment paper.
3. Drizzle olive oil over the salmon and season with salt and pepper.
4. Place lemon slices on top of the salmon fillets and sprinkle with fresh dill.
5. Bake in the preheated oven for 12-15 minutes or until the salmon flakes easily with a fork.
6. Serve the baked salmon with your favorite Paleo-friendly side dishes.

Foods to Avoid:

The main foods to eliminate are processed foods, the largest source of toxicity and malnutrition. Processed foods are the easiest items to eat

these days, and we eat entirely too much. Grains that form the base of sandwich breads, cereals and pasta have no place in the Paleo Diet. Also, the processed fats and vegetable seed oils are also counterproductive to our health. Legumes, especially soy, and vegetable seed oils should be banished from your diet. There are no refined sugars little dairy and absolutely no processed foods in the Paleo plan.

1. Processed Foods: This includes most things that come in a box, bag, or can.

2. Grains: No wheat, oats, barley, or other grains, including gluten-free options.

3. Legumes: Avoid beans, lentils, and peanuts.

4. Dairy: Most forms of dairy, including milk, cheese, and yogurt, are excluded. Some people include ghee or clarified butter.

5. Refined Sugar: This includes both white and brown sugars, as well as high-fructose corn syrup.

6. Processed Vegetable Oils: Such as soybean oil, sunflower oil, and corn oil.

7. Artificial Sweeteners and Additives: These are not considered Paleo-friendly.

 Tips for Paleo Dieting:

1. Plan Your Meals: Planning is essential to ensure you have Paleo-friendly options available.

2. Read Labels: Even seemingly healthy foods can contain non-Paleo ingredients, so always check labels.

3. Cook at Home: This gives you complete control over the ingredients in your meals.

4. Stay Hydrated: Drink plenty of water throughout the day.

5. Exercise Regularly: Combine your diet with regular physical activity for better results.

6. Listen to Your Body: Everyone's body is different. Pay attention to how different foods make you feel and adjust your diet accordingly.

7. Consult a Professional: If you have any health concerns or specific dietary needs, it's always a good idea to consult a healthcare provider or a registered dietitian.

Remember, before making any significant changes to your diet, especially if you have underlying health conditions, it's advisable to consult a healthcare professional to ensure the Paleo diet is suitable for your individual needs.

Paleo Friendly Desserts

One of the biggest stumbling blocks with the Paleo Diet plan is desserts. Most desserts have unnatural sweeteners and starchy carbs that spike insulin levels. Most sweet treats are a recipe for disaster. However, with kids, special celebrations and Birthdays sometimes a sweet treat is in order. There are some very tasty Paleo desserts that can help you transition fully into the Paleo lifestyle without indulging in bad choices or having a gluten stomach ache. While it is not a good idea to eat desserts after every meal, Paleo friendly desserts can stop hardcore cravings from your pre-Paleo days.

Here is a list of whole food substitutions you can use to whip delicious Paleo friendly desserts together.

· Almond flour- Grinding almonds create nutritious, high protein flour perfect for making muffins breads and of course, traditional macaroons.

· Raw Honey– Because honey can be eaten straight from the tree, it is considered a true Paleo sweetener. Though it is a whole food, honey is highly caloric and does spike the insulin level, so leave sparingly. However, honey is the perfect sugar substitute.

· Cocoa- Unsweetened dark chocolate has nutritious antioxidants and sticks to the limited dairy rules. Opt for the natural cocoa over the Dutch processed version that loses its benefits during processing.

· Pure Vanilla Extract– Pure vanilla extract is a staple in any baker's cupboard. Just make sure to buy the pure stuff not the cheap flavouring.

· Coconut Oil- Coconut oil is a medium chain fatty acid, which means it transfers directly to the liver where it is used for energy instead of being stored directly as fat. It also stimulates the thyroid gland helping speed up metabolism. Coconut oil adds a subtle sweetness to cobbler's pancakes and other baked recipes.

· Coconut Milk- A great dairy substitute, coconut milk contains lauric acid. Lauric acid is proven to fight influenza, herpes, HIV as well as improve the immune system. Use coconut oil to make ice cream, hot cocoa, pudding, and even egg nog.

· Nuts– Nuts are loaded with good fats the bodies need. Hazelnuts, pecans, macadamias and almonds are lifesavers in the kitchen. Use nuts for pie crusts, candies or even as simple spiced nut blend.

· Frozen Fruit- Freeze berries to make easy desserts. Use them to make rich frothy smoothies or sorbet. Frozen grapes and cherries taste delicious straight from the freezer. Try frozen bananas on a stick or blended down for a creamy ice cream experience.

· Dates- Dates are natural sweeteners that do not add its own flavour like honey.

They contain simple sugars like dextrose and fructose that are easy to digest and replenish your energy. Blend dates in the food processor with wet ingredients when baking. They also work well for binding snack bars.

Certainly! There are plenty of delicious paleo-friendly desserts you can enjoy. Here's a simple and tasty recipe for paleo-friendly chocolate avocado mousse:

Paleo Chocolate Avocado Mousse

Ingredients:

- 2 ripe avocados, peeled and pitted

- 1/4 cup unsweetened cocoa powder

- 1/4 cup almond milk (or any other paleo-friendly milk)

- 1/4 cup honey or maple syrup (adjust to taste)

- 1 teaspoon vanilla extract

- Pinch of salt

- Optional toppings: fresh berries, coconut flakes, chopped nuts

Instructions:

1. Blend Avocado: In a blender or food processor, blend the avocados until smooth and creamy.

2. Add Ingredients: Add the cocoa powder, almond milk, honey (or maple syrup), vanilla extract, and a pinch of salt to the blender. Blend until all the ingredients are well combined and the mixture is creamy.

3. Taste and Adjust: Taste the mousse and adjust the sweetness according to your preference by adding more honey or maple syrup if needed.

4. Chill: Transfer the mousse to serving glasses or bowls and refrigerate for at least 30 minutes to chill and firm up.

5. Serve: Before serving, you can garnish the mousse with fresh berries, coconut flakes, or chopped nuts for added texture and flavor.

Enjoy your creamy and indulgent chocolate avocado mousse without any guilt!

Remember, while these desserts are paleo-friendly, portion control is still essential, as they can be calorie-dense. Enjoy in moderation!

THE PALEO LIFESTYLE

Tips for the Paleo Lifestyle

Unfortunately, the cheapest and quickest foods available today are usually the least nutritious. Our busy lifestyles have our kids raised on a diet of processed and fast foods.

The popular culture even makes eating real foods an odd concept. Even knowing the proven benefits, some never try the Paleo diet because they believe it is too difficult.

Living a long, healthy fulfilling life is well worth a few small changes. While not as easy as stopping at a drive through, maintaining a Paleo lifestyle is realistic with a few tips.

· Stay Organized- The number one tip is to be organized and prepared. The biggest challenge will be to have Paleo foods available at your home and plan your meals.

You are much more likely to eat healthy food choices if it is readily available at home.

· Change how you Shop- Find the best farmers markets, butchers and grocery stores in your area. Before going to the grocery have a list of items you plan to pick up. Also, shop the perimeter of grocery stores to avoid the aisles filled with processed foods. This may be difficult at first,

but after a month or so you will no longer feel a need to peruse the sugar aisles.

· Clean your Pantry- Clear your cupboards of all the cereals, pasta, and processed foods in your cabinets. Don't worry. You will replace these foods with much more satisfying fresh and healthy foods.

· Learn to Work the Kitchen- Unlike a diet based on grains, there are many foods to eat on the Paleo Diet you should never become bored. The best way to take advantage of everything nature has to offer is to learn how to cook. By combining the diverse flavours, there is an endless amount of tasty dishes to excite your taste buds.

· Dress Your Food- Most of the condiments on the store shelves are filled with preservatives. However, you can enhance the flavour of your foods

by making your own condiments at home. Ketchup, mustard, salad dressings and sauces can be made at home naturally with delicious results.

· Exercise- Just changing your eating habits will cause you to lose weight naturally on the Paleo Diet. Add exercise to the mix, and you will be amazed at how quickly you notice a difference. Your true, toned physique will come out as pounds shed.

You will also notice the amount of energy increased compared to when you ate a traditional diet. Start feeling strong, energetic, and mentally sharper and all round younger.

· Join Support System, find chat rooms and forums where like-minded people meet. Participate at a gym where the Paleo Diet is the main lifestyle choice. It is nice to share ideas on the best Paleo books, and even give advice on keeping true to the diet plan. Joining a community online

or in person is extremely motivating when you learn about how the other member's lives improved just from staying true to the Paleo way.

CONCLUSION

The Paleo Diet is proven to shed pounds and have a healthier life. Add exercise to the mix and you can achieve the lean, sexy bodies seen on fitness models. Despite popular belief, the Paleo lifestyle is not restrictive and can actually open your palette to a whole new world of culinary experiences. There are a variety of high quality cookbooks and website

that will help you along the way. Once you experience the transformation you will wonder how you ever functioned. Get the most of your life and enjoy optimum fitness with the Paleo diet plan.